3103 3078   8/04

The All Natural
Facial Recipe Book

The All Natural Facial Recipe Book

Dawn M. Waldock

NEW CENTURY BOOKS

New Century Books
P.O. Box 1205
Santa Teresa, N.M. 88008
2002114508
Library of Congress number

ISBN 0-930751-54-X Hardcover
ISBN 0-930751-55-8 Paperback

****

Thank you

****

To my husband, Gary
Thank you
For helping to make
My dreams come true.
I love you.

Tons

I thank my family and friends
for supporting and believing in me
and allowing me to slather them
with these recipes time after time.

Thank you soooo much.

****

Contents

****

****

Introduction

The all natural facial recipe book offers organic alternatives to synthetic substances. Many commercial products contain chemicals that can be harmful to our skin.

Now you can use all natural readily available ingredients that you may have in your kitchen to create your own natural facial recipes.

Important

****

Always do a patch test before using any of these recipes.

To do the patch test, apply a little bit of the recipe to the inside elbow and leave for 24 hours. If there is reddening, itching or other adverse side effects, do not use. Consult a physician or dermatologist before proceeding. If you know you are allergic to an item do not use.

The eye area should be avoided with all the recipes in this book.

Always use clean equipment and ingredients

****

Note

Shelf Life

****

The recipes in this book are intended to be made fresh with every use. If keeping the remainder of a recipe, cover and refrigerate immediately; discard after 1 day.

None of the recipes are intended for internal use so if placing in refrigerator mark container accordingly.

The eye area should be avoided with all the recipes in this book.

Always use clean equipment and ingredients

****

Vegetarian Substitutions

****

Soymilk for milk
Soymilk for yogurt
Corn syrup for Honey

****

Allergy substitutions

****

If you are allergic to an item in the recipe do not use it.

Substitute something else you are not allergic to that does the same thing. A glossary is in the back of the book for some ideas.

****

Dawn M. Waldock

Skin Types

****

Oily: If your skin secretes a lot of sebum. It gives a shiny appearance and is prone to acne and blackheads.

Dry: This skin type is the opposite of oily. The skin lacks sebum which protects and keeps skin moist. The result may be dry flaky skin.

Combination: This is the most common skin type now. It is a combination of oily and dry skin

Normal: Few people have normal skin. If your skin is not dry or oily then it is normal.

Sensitive: Dry, fine and prone to rash and allergies

****

Conversion Chart

****

Dry

3 teaspoons = 1 tablespoons
4 tablespoons = 1/4 cup =2 ounces

****

Liquid

1/4 cup = 2fluid ounces
Fresh lemon = about 3 tablespoons
Fresh orange = about 1/3 cup

****

The Five Step Face Plan

****

Cleanse: *To free the skin of dirt, oil and makeup*

Steam: *To open the pores for deep -cleansing (once a week)*

Mask: *To cleanse deep within the pores*

Tone: *To tighten the pores*

Moisturize: *To replenish and protect the skin*

****

Cleansers and Scrubs

****

Facial masks can be used on all skin types, for a variety of reasons; They can remove excess oil from the skin, they can tighten pores or they can moisturize and replenish dry skin. All masks may not be right for your skin type.

**Avoid the eye area
with cleansers and scrubs**

Don't forget your neck.

Remember to do your patch test.

****

Oats Facial Cleanser

For All Skin Types

****

1/4 cup ground oats
1/4 cup plain yogurt

****

Combine ingredients together to form a paste. Apply the mixture directly to the skin. Remove by very gently rubbing with warm water and using your finger tips in a circular motion. Follow with a cool water rinse and then gently pat dry.

Oats: Cleanser, exfoliant
Yogurt: Moisturizer, exfoliant

Remember to do your patch test.

****

The Quickie Wash

For All Skin Types

****

1 tablespoon distilled water
1 tablespoon apple cider vinegar

****

In a small bowl combine both ingredients.
Mix and apply to the face with a cotton ball.
(avoid the eye area). Follow with a cool
water rinse and then gently pat dry.

Distilled Water: Dilutes
Apple Cider Vinegar: Acts as Astringent and
oil remover

Remember to do your patch test.

****

The Quickie Cleaner

For All Skin Types

****

1/8 cup honey

****

Apply to the face, leave on 5 minutes (avoid the eye area). Remove with warm water. Follow with a cool water rinse and then gently pat dry.

Honey: Moisturizer, exfoliant

Remember to do your patch test.

****

Almond Paste Scrub

For Normal Skin

****

1/4 cup ground almonds
2 tablespoons honey
2 tablespoons milk

****

Grind almonds in mini food processor.
Combine all ingredients together to form a
paste. Apply the mixture directly to the skin.
Remove by very gently rubbing with warm
water and using your finger tips in a circular motion. Follow with a cool water rinse
and then gently pat dry.

Ground almonds: Cleanser, exfoliant
Honey: Moisturizer, exfoliant
Milk: Cleanser, emollient

Remember to do your patch test.

****

Alfalfa and Almond Scrub

For Normal Skin

****

4 tablespoons chopped alfalfa sprouts
1/4 cup ground almonds
2 tablespoons honey

****

Grind almonds in mini food processor. Combine all ingredients together to form a paste. Apply the mixture directly to the skin. Remove by very gently rubbing with warm water and using your finger tips in a circular motion. Follow with a cool water rinse and then gently pat dry.

Alfalfa Sprouts: Astringent
Ground almonds: Cleanser, exfoliant
Honey: Moisturizer, exfoliant

Remember to do your patch test.

****

Cornstarch Cleanser

For Normal Skin

****

2 tablespoons cornstarch
1 tablespoon milk
1 tablespoon yogurt

****

Mix all ingredients together. Apply directly to the skin, avoiding the eye area. Leave on face for 3 minutes gently massage in circular motions while rinsing with cool water, then gently pat dry.

Cornstarch: Cleanser, exfoliant
Milk: Emollient, cleanser
Yogurt: Moisturizer, exfoliant

Remember to do your patch test.

****

Baking Soda Scrub

For Normal Skin

****

2 tablespoons baking soda
1 tablespoon yogurt
2 teaspoons lemon juice

****

Combine all ingredients together to form a paste. Apply the mixture directly to the skin. Remove by very gently rubbing with warm water and using your finger tips in a circular motion. Follow with a cool water rinse and then gently pat dry.

Baking Soda: Cleanser, exfoliant
Yogurt: Cleanser, emollient
Lemon juice: Exfoliant, astringent

Remember to do your patch test.

****

Cornmeal Cleanser

For Oily Skin

****

1/2 cup cornmeal
1/4 cup plain yogurt
3-4 fresh mint leaves

****

Mix cornmeal and yogurt together. Add fresh chopped mint leaves. Apply directly to the skin, avoiding the eye area. Leave on face for 3 minutes gently massage in circular motions while rinsing with cool water, then gently pat dry.

Cornmeal: Cleanser, exfoliant
Yogurt: Moisturizer, exfoliant
Mint leaves: Refresher, stimulant

Remember to do your patch test.

****

Cider Vinegar Cleanser

For Oily Skin

****

2 tablespoons apple cider vinegar
4 tablespoons distilled water
3-4 fresh mint leaves

****

Mix vinegar and water together. Add fresh finely chopped mint leaves. Apply directly to the skin with a cotton ball, avoiding the eye area. Rinse with Tepid water, and then gently pat dry.

Apple cider vinegar: Oil remover
Distilled water: Dilute vinegar
Mint leaves: Refresher, stimulant

Remember to do your patch test.

****

Apple and Pine Nut Cleanser

For Oily Skin

****

1/4 cup pine nuts
1/8 cup apple
3 tablespoons yogurt
1 teaspoon fresh lemon juice

****

Blend all ingredients together in a mini-food processor. Apply to face. Massage gently with an outward circular motion avoiding the eye area. Rinse with cool water, and then gently pat dry.

Pine nuts: Cleanser, exfoliant
Yogurt: Moisturizer, exfoliant
Apple: Exfoliant
Lemon juice: Astringent, oil remover

Remember to do your patch test.

****

Pine Nut Cleanser

For Oily Skin

****

1/8 cup pine nuts
1 tablespoons honey

****

Blend pine nuts in a mini-food processor or coffee grinder. Add ground nuts to honey. Apply to face. Massage gently with an outward circular motion avoiding the eye area. Rinse with cool water, and then gently pat dry.

Pine nuts: Cleanser, exfoliant
Honey: Moisturizer, exfoliant

Remember to do your patch test.

****

Papaya Sesame Seed Scrub

For Oily Skin

****

1/4 cup chopped papaya
1/4 cup sesame seeds
1/4 cup plain yogurt
2 tablespoons honey

****

Blend all ingredients together in a mini food processor except the sesame seeds. Combine all ingredients together, gently massage in circular motions rinsing with cool water and gently pat dry.

Sesame seeds: Cleanser, exfoliant
Papaya: Exfoliant
Yogurt: Moisturizer, exfoliant
Honey: Humectant, emollient

Remember to do your patch test.

****

Honey Oat Scrub

For Oily Skin

****

1/4 cup ground oats
2 tablespoons honey
1 tablespoon plain yogurt
1 tablespoon finely chopped parsley

****

Mix all the ingredients together. Apply to the face. Leave on 15 minutes. Remove by very gently rubbing with warm water and using your finger tips. Follow with a cool water rinse and then gently pat dry.

Oats: Cleanser, exfoliant
Honey: Humectant, emollient
Yogurt: Moisturizer, exfoliant
Parsley: Cleanser, soother, Healant

Remember to do your patch test.

****

Alfalfa and Oats Scrub

For Dry Skin

****

4 tablespoons chopped alfalfa
1/4 cup ground oats
1 egg yolk

****

Mix all the ingredients together. Apply to the face. Leave on 15 minutes. Remove by very gently rubbing using your finger tips. Rinse with warm water. Follow with a cool water rinse and then gently pat dry.

Alfalfa: Astringent, soothes
Oats: Cleanser, exfoliant
Egg yolk: Toner, conditioner

Remember to do your patch test.

****

Sesame Seed Scrub

For Dry Skin

****

1/4 cup sesame seeds
1 egg yolk
2 tablespoons honey
1 tablespoon plain yogurt

****

Mix all the ingredients together. Apply to the face. Leave on face 15 minutes. Remove by very gently rubbing using your finger tips. Rinse with warm water. Follow with a cool water rinse and then gently pat dry.

Sesame seeds: Cleanser, exfoliant
Egg yolk: Toner, conditioner
Honey: Humectant, emollient
Yogurt: Moisturizer, exfoliant

Remember to do your patch test.

****

Honey Cornmeal Scrub

For Dry Skin

****

1/4 cup cornmeal
1 tablespoon milk
1 tablespoon honey
4 mashed seedless grapes

****

Mix all the ingredients together. Apply to the face. Leave on 15 minutes. Remove by very gently rubbing using your finger tips. Rinse with warm water. Follow with a cool water rinse and then gently pat dry.

Cornmeal: Cleanser, exfoliant
Milk: Cleanser, moisturizer
Honey: Humectant, emollient
Grapes: Anti-inflammatory

Remember to do your patch test.

****

Pesto Scrub

For Dry Skin

****

1/4 cup basil
2 tablespoons pine nuts
1 tablespoon honey
1 tablespoon olive oil

****

Blend pine nuts, basil and olive oil in a mini food processor or blender then add honey. Apply to the face. Remove by very gently rubbing using your finger tips. Rinse with warm water then cool water then gently pat dry.

Basil: Pain reliever, stimulant
Pine nuts: Conditioner, softener
Honey: Humectant, emollient
Olive oil: Conditioner

Remember to do your patch test.

****

Pineapple Scrub
For Dry Skin

****

1/4 cup chopped fresh pineapple
2 tablespoons yogurt
1 tablespoon honey
1 tablespoon olive oil

****

Blend peeled cut pineapple in a mini food processor or blender then add honey, yogurt and olive oil. Apply to the face gently in a circular outward motion with finger tips. Rinse with warm water then with cool water then gently pat dry.

Pineapple Exfoliant, soother
Yogurt: Emollient, exfoliant
Honey: Humectant, emollient
Olive oil: Conditioner

Remember to do your patch test.

****

Sesame Honey Scrub

For Dry Skin

****

1/8 cup sesame seeds
3 tablespoons honey

****

Combine all ingredients together Apply to the
face. Gently massage in circular motion,
rinse with cool water and gently pat dry.

Sesame seeds: Cleanser, exfoliant
Honey: Humectant, emollient

Remember to do your patch test.

****

Creamy Cucumber Cleanser
For Sensitive Skin

****

1/4 cup chopped cucumber
3 tablespoons yogurt

****

Puree seeded chopped cucumber in a blender
Add cucumber to yogurt and Apply to the
face. Gently massage in circular motion.
Rinse with cool water and gently pat dry.

Cucumber: Cleanser, exfoliant
Yogurt: Emollient, exfoliant

Remember to do your patch test.

****

Oatmeal Facial Cleanser

For Sensitive Skin

****

1/4 cup ground oats
1 tablespoon distilled water

****

Chop oatmeal in a coffee grinder. Remove
and mix ingredients together to form a
paste. Apply the mixture directly to the skin.
Remove by very gently rubbing with warm
water and using your finger tips in a circular motion. Follow with a cool water rinse
and then gently pat dry.

Oats: Cleanser, exfoliant
Distilled water: Dilute

Remember to do your patch test.

****

Facial Steam

 A Facial steam can be used on all skin types. Facial steams deep-cleanse your skin. Gently steaming the skin aids in circulation and eliminating toxins. All steams may not be right for your skin type. Always clean your face before doing a steam.

Normal skin: steam weekly
Oily skin: steam twice weekly
Dry skin: every other week

Do not do a facial steam if you have a serious skin problem without first checking with your physician.

Remember to do your patch test.

****

Rose Petal Steam

For All Skin Types

****

3 cups of distilled water
1/4 rose petals

****

Boil water. Remove it from the heat before adding the rose petals. Let steep for 5 minutes, use a towel over your head and shoulders to create a tent. Lean over pot (at least 12 inches above). Close your eyes, breathe and relax. Be careful not to spill. It is hot.

Distilled Water: Dilute
Rose petals: Astringent, toner

Remember to do your patch test.

****

Chamomile Tea Steam

For Dry Skin

****

1 chamomile tea bag
3 cups of distilled water
1 tablespoon chopped mint

****

Boil water. Remove from heat before adding the mint and tea bag. Remove from heat. Let steep for 10 minutes use a towel over your head and shoulders to create a tent, And then lean over pot (at least 12 inches above). Close your eyes, breathe and relax. Be careful not to spill. It is hot.

Chamomile tea: Healant
Distilled water: For the steam
Mint: Stimulant, refresher

Remember to do your patch test.

****

Distilled Water Steam

For All Skin Types

****

4 cups of distilled water

****

Boil water. Remove from heat. Let cool 3-5 minutes. Use a towel over your head and shoulders to create a tent. Lean over pot (at least 12 inches above). Close your eyes, breathe and relax. Be careful not to spill. It is hot.

Distilled Water: Open pores, for the steam

Remember to do your patch test.

****

Sage Steam

For oily Skin

****

4 cups of distilled water
2 tablespoons dried sage

****

Boil water. Remove it from the heat before adding the dried sage. Let steep for 5 minutes. Use a towel over your head and shoulders to create a tent. Lean over pot (at least 12 inches above). Close your eyes, breathe and relax. Be careful not to spill. It is hot.

Distilled Water: For the steam
Sage: Astringent, toner

Remember to do your patch test.

****

Catnip Steam

For oily Skin

****

4 cups of distilled water
2 tablespoons dried catnip

****

Boil water. Remove it from the heat before adding the dried catnip. Let steep for 5 minutes, use a towel over your head and shoulders to create a tent. Lean over pot (at least 12 inches above). Close your eyes, breathe and relax. Be careful not to spill. It is hot.

Distilled Water: For the steam
Catnip: Astringent, toner

Remember to do your patch test.

****

Basil Steam

For oily Skin

****

4 cups of distilled water
2 tablespoons dried basil

****

Boil water. Remove it from the heat before adding the dried basil. Let steep for 5 minutes. Use a towel over your head and shoulders to create a tent. Lean over pot (at least 12 inches above). Close your eyes, breathe and relax. Be careful not to spill. It is hot.

Distilled Water: For the steam
Basil: Soother, stimulant

Remember to do your patch test.

****

Rosemary Steam

For oily Skin

****

4 cups of distilled water
2 tablespoons dried rosemary

****

Boil water. Remove it from the heat before adding the dried rosemary. Let steep for 5 minutes, use a towel over your head and shoulders to create a tent. Lean over pot (at least 12 inches above). Close your eyes, breathe and relax. Be careful not to spill. It is hot.

Distilled Water: For the steam dilute
Rosemary: Astringent, stimulant

Remember to do your patch test.

****

Mint Steam

For oily Skin

****

4 cups of distilled water
2 tablespoons dried mint

****

Boil water. Remove it from the heat before
adding the dried mint. Let steep for 5
minutes. Use a towel over your head and
shoulders to create a tent. Lean over pot
(at least 12 inches above). Close your eyes,
breathe and relax. Be careful not to spill.
It is hot.

Distilled Water: For the steam dilute
Mint: Astringent, stimulant

Remember to do your patch test.

****

Facial Masks

Facial masks can be used on all skin types, for a variety of reasons. They can remove excess oil from the skin, they can tighten pores or they can moisturize and replenish dry skin All masks may not be right for your skin type.

Remember to do your patch test.

Egg and Beer Mask

For All Skin Types

****

1 egg white
1 tablespoon plain yogurt
2 tablespoons beer
1 teaspoon olive oil

****

In a Blender Mix all the ingredients together. Apply to the face. Leave on the face 15 minutes. Remove with warm water. Follow with a cool water rinse and then gently pat dry.

Egg white: Toner, conditioner
Beer: Skin softener, soother
Yogurt: Moisturizer, exfoliant
Olive oil: Conditioner, softener

Remember to do your patch test.

****

Honey and Egg Mask

For Normal Skin

****

1 egg white
2 tablespoons honey
1 tablespoon plain yogurt

****

Mix all the ingredients together. Apply to the face. Leave on face 15 minutes. Remove with warm water. Follow with a cool water rinse and then gently pat dry.

Egg white: Toner, conditioner
Honey: Humectant, emollient
Yogurt: Moisturizer, exfoliant

Remember to do your patch test.

****

Orange Yogurt Mask

For Normal Skin

****

1 tablespoon orange juice
3 tablespoons yogurt

****

Juice an orange. Add yogurt. Apply to the face and leave on 5-10 minutes. Rinse with warm water then with cool water then gently pat dry.

Orange juice: Astringent, exfoliant
Yogurt: Moisturizer, exfoliant

Remember to do your patch test.

****

Cucumber and Yogurt Mask

For Normal Skin

****

1/2 cucumber
2 tablespoons plain yogurt

****

Peel the cucumber and slice in half length-
wise. Remove the seeds, and then combine all
the ingredients in a blender or a small food
processor until smooth. Apply to the face and
leave on 20-30 minutes. Rinse with cool water
then gently pat dry.

Cucumber: Astringent, refresher
Yogurt: Moisturizer, exfoliant

Remember to do your patch test.

****

Milk and Honey Mask

For Normal Skin

****

4 tablespoons honey
1 tablespoon milk
1 egg white

****

Mix all the ingredients together. Apply to the face. Leave on 20-30 minutes. Remove with wash cloth soaked in warm water. Follow with a cool water rinse and then gently pat dry.

Honey: Humectant, emollient
Milk: Cleanser, emollient
Egg white: Toner, conditioner

Remember to do your patch test.

****

Peach and Honey Mask

For Normal Skin

****

1 medium fresh peach
2 tablespoons honey
3 tablespoons oatmeal

****

Peel and cut a fresh peach. Mash with a fork, add honey and oatmeal. Should be a thick consistency (add more oatmeal if needed). Apply to the face and leave on 10-15 minutes. Rinse well with cool water, then gently pat dry.

Peach: Conditioner, soother
Honey: Humectant, emollient
Oatmeal: Cleanser, exfoliant

Remember to do your patch test.

****

Lemon and Honey Mask

For Normal Skin

****

4 tablespoons honey
1 tablespoon lemon juice

****

Mix all the ingredients together. Apply to the face. Leave on 20-30 minutes. Remove with wash cloth soaked in warm water. Follow with a cool water rinse and then gently pat dry.

Honey: Humectant, emollient
Lemon juice: Astringent, oil remover

Remember to do your patch test.

****

Peel Off Mask

For Normal Skin

****

2 tablespoon unflavored gelatin
3 tablespoons milk

****

Mix the ingredients together. Microwave
mask for10-15 seconds. Apply to the face.
Leave on 20-30 minutes. Peel off when dried
completely.

Gelatin: Fortifier
Milk: Cleanser, emollient

Remember to do your patch test.

****

Strawberry Facial Recipe
For Oily Skin

****

8 fresh whole strawberries
3 tablespoons honey

****

Use a fork mash strawberries into a pulp, then add honey. Mix. (Do not over mix or it will be runny). Apply directly to the skin, leave on for 3-5 minutes. Rinse with warm water and then with cool water. Gently pat dry.

Strawberries: Cleanser, exfoliant
Honey: Humectant, emollient

Remember to do your patch test.

****

Apple Facial Mask

For Oily Skin

****

1/2 apple grated
6 tablespoons honey

****

Mix grated apple and honey together. Smooth over skin and let sit for 5-10 minutes. Rinse with warm water and then with cool water. Gently pat dry.

Apple: Exfoliant, oil remover
Honey: Humectant, emollient

Remember to do your patch test.

****

Lemon and Egg Mask
For Oily Skin

****

1/2 fresh lemon
1 egg white

****

Squeeze 1/2 a lemon (no seeds)
Beat the lemon and egg white together for 3 minutes, smooth over skin and let sit for 15 - 20 minutes. Avoid the eye area. Rinse with warm water and then with cool water. Gently pat dry. Follow with a moisturizer.

Egg white: Toner, ingredient binder
Lemon juice: Astringent, oil remover

Remember to do your patch test.

****

Carrot Facial Mask

For Oily Skin

****

2 large carrots
4 tablespoons honey
1 tablespoon plain yogurt

****

Cook carrots, then mash. Mix with honey and yogurt. Apply gently to the skin. After 10 minutes rinse with warm water then with cool water. Gently pat dry.

Carrots: Healant, exfoliant
Honey: Humectant, emollient
Yogurt: Moisturizer, exfoliant

Remember to do your patch test.

****

Strawberry and Yogurt Mask

For Oily Skin

****

4 strawberries
1 tablespoon honey
1/4 cup plain yogurt

****

Mash strawberries. Mix with honey and yogurt. Apply gently to the skin. After 10-15 minutes rinse with warm water and then with cool water. Gently pat dry.

Strawberries: Cleanser, exfoliant
Honey: Humectant, emollient
Yogurt: Moisturizer, exfoliant

Remember to do your patch test.

****

Strawberry Mint Mask

For Oily Skin

****

8 strawberries
1 tablespoon mint
1 tablespoon plain yogurt

****

Mash strawberries. Mix with freshly chopped mint and yogurt. Apply gently to the skin. After 10-15 minutes rinse with warm water and then with cool water. Gently pat dry.

Strawberries: Cleanser, exfoliant
Mint: Astringent, antiseptic, toner
Yogurt: Moisturizer, exfoliant

Remember to do your patch test.

****

Tomato Yogurt Mask

For Oily Skin

****

1/4 tomato
1/4 cup plain yogurt
3 tablespoons honey

****

Puree tomato in a blender.
Mix all the ingredients together. Apply to the face. Leave on 15 minutes. Remove with warm water and then with cool water. Gently pat dry.

Tomato: Astringent, refresher
Yogurt: Moisturizer, exfoliant
Honey: Humectant, emollient

Remember to do your patch test.

****

Tomato Mask

For Oily Skin

****

1/4 tomato
1/4 cup honey
1 tablespoon plain yogurt
1 tablespoon ground oatmeal

****

Puree tomato in a blender or food processor. Combine all the ingredients together. Apply to the face. Leave on 10-15 minutes. Remove with warm water, follow with a cool water rinse and then gently pat dry.

Tomato: Astringent, refresher
Honey: Humectant, emollient
Yogurt: Moisturizer, exfoliant
Oatmeal: Cleanser, exfoliant

Remember to do your patch test.

****

Apple Egg Mask
For Oily Skin

****

1/2 apple grated
4 tablespoons honey
2 egg whites

****

Whip egg whites. Add grated apple and honey to egg mixture. Smooth over skin and let sit for 15-20 minutes. Rinse with warm water and then with cool water. Gently pat dry.

Apple: Exfoliant, oil remover
Honey: Humectant, emollient
Egg whites: Toner, emulsifier

Remember to do your patch test.

****

Cucumber and Egg Mask

For Dry Skin

****

1/4 cucumber
2 egg yolks
2 tablespoons honey
2 tablespoons ground oats

****

Peel and remove the seeds from the cucumber, add all ingredients to a small food processor and blend for 1 minute. Apply to the face and leave 15 minutes. Rinse with warm water then with cool water gently pat dry.

Cucumber: Astringent, refresher
Egg Yolk: Toner, emulsifier
Honey: Humectant, emollient
Oatmeal: Cleanser, exfoliant

Remember to do your patch test.

****

Banana Facial Mask
For Dry Skin

****

1 banana
2 tablespoons honey
2 tablespoons ground oats

****

Mash banana with a fork. Don't over mash or it will be too runny. Add honey and ground oats. Apply to the face and leave on 15 minutes. Rinse with warm water then with cool water. Gently pat dry.

Banana: Moisturizer, humectant
Honey: Humectant, emollient
Oatmeal: Cleanser, exfoliant

Remember to do your patch test.

****

Avocado and Honey Mask
For Dry Skin

****

1/4 cup avocado
2 tablespoons honey
1 egg yolk

****

Mash avocado, mix with honey and egg yolk
Apply to the face and leave on 15 minutes.
Rinse with warm water and then with cool
water. Gently pat dry.

Avocado: Moisturizer, emollient
Honey: Humectant, emollient
Egg Yolk: Toner, emulsifier

Remember to do your patch test.

****

Avocado and Yogurt Mask

For Dry Skin

****

1/4 cup avocado
2 tablespoons yogurt
2 tablespoon ground oatmeal

****

Mash avocado, mix with yogurt and oatmeal. Apply to the face and leave on 15 minutes. Rinse with warm water and then with cool water. Gently pat dry.

Avocado: Moisturizer, emollient
Yogurt: Moisturizer, exfoliant
Oatmeal: Cleanser, exfoliant

Remember to do your patch test.

****

Cucumber Avocado Mask

For Dry Skin

****

1/2 cucumber
1/2 avocado
1 egg yolk
1 tablespoon plain yogurt

****

Peel and remove the seeds from the cucumber, combine all the ingredients in a small food processor until smooth. Apply to the face and leave on 20 minutes. Rinse with warm water and then with cool water. Gently pat dry.

Cucumber: Astringent, refresher
Avocado: Moisturizer, emollient
Egg Yolk: Toner, emulsifier
Yogurt: Moisturizer, exfoliant

Remember to do your patch test.

****

Peach and Yogurt Mask
For Dry Skin

****

1 fresh peach
3 tablespoons honey
3 tablespoon plain yogurt

****

Peel and cut a fresh peach. Mash with a fork and then combine all the ingredients in a blender or a small food processor until smooth. Apply to the face and leave on 15-20 minutes. Rinse with warm water and then with cool water. Gently pat dry.

Peach: Conditioner, soother
Honey: Humectant, emollient
Yogurt: Moisturizer, exfoliant

Remember to do your patch test.

****

Banana Yogurt Mask

For Dry Skin

****

1 banana
3 tablespoons yogurt
1 tablespoons honey

****

Mash banana with a fork. Don't over mash or it will be too runny. Add honey and yogurt. Apply to the face and leave on 15 minutes. Rinse with warm water and then with cool water. Gently pat dry.

Banana: Moisturizer
Yogurt: Moisturizer, exfoliant
Honey: Humectant, emollient

Remember to do your patch test.

****

Papaya Mask

For Dry Skin

****

1/4 fresh papaya
4 tablespoons honey
2 tablespoons yogurt

****

Mash fresh papaya with a fork. Add honey.
Smooth over skin and let sit for 10 minutes.
Rinse with warm water, and then with cool
water. Gently pat dry.

Papaya: Exfoliant
Honey: Humectant, emollient
Yogurt: Yogurt: Moisturizer, exfoliant

Remember to do your patch test.

****

Papaya Peel

For Dry Skin

****

1/2 fresh papaya
1 packet unflavored gelatin
2 tablespoons distilled water

****

In saucepan combine water and gelatin, dissolve over low heat. Cut and peel papaya, then blend thoroughly in a blender. Strain and keep liquid. In a small bowl combine gelatin and papaya juice Refrigerate for 15 minutes spread over face 20minutes. Rinse with wash cloth and warm water and then gently pat dry.

Papaya: Exfoliant
Distilled Water: Dilutes
Gelatin: Thickens

Remember to do your patch test.

****

Banana and Peach Mask
For Dry Skin

****

1/2 banana
1/2 peach
2 tablespoons honey
2 tablespoons yogurt

****

Mash banana and peach with a fork. (Don't over mash or it will be too runny.) Add honey and yogurt. Apply to the face and leave on 10-15 minutes. Rinse with warm water then with cool water. Gently pat dry.

Banana: moisturizer
Peach: Conditioner, soother
Honey: Humectant, emollient
Yogurt: Yogurt: Moisturizer, exfoliant

Remember to do your patch test.

****

Pesto Mask

For Dry Skin

****

1/4 cup basil
1 tablespoons honey
2 tablespoons olive oil

****

Blend basil and olive oil in a mini food processor or blender then add honey Apply to the face and leave on 10-15 minutes. Rinse with warm water then with cool water. Gently pat dry.

Honey: Humectant, emollient
Olive oil: Conditioner
Basil: Pain reliever, stimulant

Remember to do your patch test.

****

Facial Toners

****

Facial toners usually contain some kind of astringent to tighten the pores. The most common is lemon because of the pleasant smell. Vinegar, witch hazel and egg are other popular toners.

Remember to do your patch test.

****

Rose Water

For Normal Skin

****

1/2 cup Rose petals
1/2 cup distilled water

****

Bring water to a boil and pour over rose petals and let steep for 30 minutes. Strain the petals and Apply liquid to face using a cotton ball. Rinse with cool water.

Distilled water: For distillation
Rose Petals: Emollient

Avoid the eye area

Remember to do your patch test.

****

Chamomile Tea Toner

For Normal Skin

****

2 chamomile tea bags
1/2 distilled water
1 tablespoon lemon juice

****

Bring Water to a boil. Add Chamomile Tea and steep for 1/2 hour. Remove Tea bags and stir in lemon juice. Apply to face using a cotton ball. Rinse with cool water.

Chamomile tea bag: Soother, healer
Distilled Water: For distillation
Lemon Juice: Astringent, toner

Avoid the eye area

Remember to do your patch test.

****

Alfalfa Grape Toner

For Normal Skin

****

12 seedless grapes
1/4 cup alfalfa sprouts
1/2 cup distilled water

****

Blend all the ingredients together in a food processor making sure everything is blended well. Strain, then apply to face using a cotton ball. Rinse with cool water.

Grapes: Soother
Lemon Juice: Astringent, Toner
Distilled Water: Dilute

Avoid the eye area

Remember to do your patch test.

****

Orange Milk Toner

For Normal Skin

****

1/2 cup milk
4 tablespoons fresh orange juice
1 tablespoon fresh lemon juice

****

Simmer milk. Remove from heat. Add orange and lemon juice let steep for 15 minutes and then strain. After cooling. Apply liquid to face using a cotton ball. Rinse with cool water.

Milk: Cleanser, emollient
Orange juice: Astringent, Toner
Lemon juice: Astringent, oil remover

Avoid the eye area

Remember to do your patch test.

****

Lime Mint Toner

For Oily Skin

****

1/4 cup distilled water
1 tablespoon lime juice
1 tablespoon chopped fresh mint

****

Mix the ingredients together making sure everything is blended well. Strain, then apply liquid to face using a cotton ball. Rinse with cool water.

Distilled water: Dilute
Lime: Astringent, refresher
Mint: Stimulant

Avoid the eye area

Remember to do your patch test.

****

Lemon Facial Toner

For Oily Skin

****

1/3 cup witch hazel
1/2 cup distilled water
1/3 cup lemon juice

****

Mix the ingredients together making sure
everything is blended well. Apply liquid to
face with a cotton ball. Rinse with cool water.

Witch Hazel: Antiseptic, astringent
Distilled water: Dilute
Lemon juice: Astringent, toner

Avoid the eye area

Remember to do your patch test.

****

Watermelon Toner

For Oily Skin

****

2 tablespoons watermelon juice
3 tablespoon distilled water
3 tablespoons witch hazel

****

Blend Watermelon in a food processor (no Peel) making sure everything is blended well. Strain and use the liquid. Add the remaining ingredients. Apply liquid to face using a cotton ball. Rinse with cool water.

Watermelon: Astringent, toner
Distilled water: Dilute
Apple Cider Vinegar: Astringent

Avoid the eye area

Remember to do your patch test.

****

Lemon and Apple Toner
For Oily Skin

****

2 tablespoons lemon juice
1/2 apple
1/2 cup distilled water

****

Blend all the ingredients together in a food processor making sure everything is blended well. Strain and then apply liquid to face using a cotton ball. Rinse with cool water.

Apple: Astringent
Distilled water: Dilute
Lemon juice: Astringent, toner

Avoid the eye area

Remember to do your patch test.

****

Orange Toner

For Oily Skin

****

2 tablespoons orange juice
3 tablespoons witch hazel
3 tablespoons distilled water

****

Blend all the ingredients together making sure everything is blended well. Apply liquid to face using a cotton ball. Rinse with cool water.

Orange juice: Astringent
Witch hazel: Antiseptic, astringent
Distilled water: Dilute

Avoid the eye area

Remember to do your patch test.

****

Grapefruit Toner
For Oily Skin

****

2 tablespoons grapefruit juice
3 tablespoons witch hazel
3 tablespoons distilled water

****

Blend all the ingredients together making sure everything is blended well. Apply liquid to face using a cotton ball. Rinse with cool water.

Grapefruit juice: Astringent
Witch hazel: Antiseptic, astringent
Distilled water: Dilute

Avoid the eye area

Remember to do your patch test.

****

Rose Rosemary Toner
For Oily Skin

****

1/2 cup witch hazel
1 small sprig of rosemary
Rose petals from 1 dried rose
1/2 cup distilled water

****

Mix the ingredients together making sure everything is blended well. Strain and then apply liquid to face using a cotton ball. Rinse with cool water.

Witch Hazel: Antiseptic, Astringent
Rosemary: Stimulant, Astringent
Rose Petals: Softener, mild cleanser
Distilled water: Dilute

Avoid the eye area

Remember to do your patch test.

****

Tomato Cucumber Toner

For Oily Skin

****

1/2 tomato
1/2 cucumber
1/8 cup vodka

****

Blend all the ingredients together in a food processor (make sure everything is blended well). Strain mixture. Apply liquid to face using a cotton ball. Rinse with cool water.

Tomato: Astringent, refresher
Cucumber: Astringent, Toner
Vodka: astringent

Avoid the eye area

Remember to do your patch test.

****

Parsley Toner

For Dry Skin

****

1/2 cup distilled water
1/4 cup chopped parsley

****

Boil water. Remove from heat. Add chopped parsley. Let steep for 15 minutes, then strain and let cool. Apply to the skin using a cotton ball. Rinse with cool water.

Distilled water: Dilute
Parsley: Astringent, toner

Avoid the eye area

Remember to do your patch test.

****

Cantaloupe Toner

For Dry Skin

****

1/2 cup distilled water
1/2 cup chopped cantaloupe
2 tablespoons witch hazel

****

Blend Cantaloupe in a food processor making sure everything is blended well. Add water and witch hazel Strain and use the liquid. Apply to the face using a cotton ball. Rinse with cool water.

Distilled water: Dilute
Cantaloupe: Refresher
Witch hazel: Antiseptic, Astringent

Avoid the eye area

Remember to do your patch test.

****

Apple Cucumber Toner

For Dry Skin

****

1/2 apple
1/2 cucumber
1/2 cup distilled water
2 tablespoons lemon juice

****

Puree all the ingredients together in a food processor (make sure everything is blended well), then strain. Use a cotton ball to apply to face. Rinse with cool water

Apple: Astringent
Cucumber: Astringent, toner
Distilled water: Dilute
Lemon juice: Astringent, toner

Avoid the eye area

Remember to do your patch test.

****

Cucumber Toner

For Dry Skin

****

1/2 cucumber
1/8 cup distilled water
1/8 cup apple cider vinegar

****

Blend all the ingredients together in a food processor (make sure everything is blended well), then strain. Use a cotton ball to apply to face. Rinse with cool water.

Cucumber: Astringent, toner
Distilled water: Dilute
Apple Cider Vinegar: Astringent

Avoid the eye area

Remember to do your patch test.

****

Grape and Cucumber Toner

For Dry Skin

****

8 seedless grapes
1/2 cucumber
1/8 cup distilled water
1/8 cup apple cider vinegar

****

Blend all the ingredients together in a food processor (make sure is everything blended well), and then strain. Use a cotton ball to apply liquid to face.

Grapes: Anti-inflammatory, soother
Cucumber: Astringent, toner
Distilled water: Dilute
Apple Cider Vinegar: astringent

Avoid the eye area

Remember to do your patch test.

****

Pineapple Toner

For Dry Skin

****

1/2 cup fresh cut pineapple
1/8 cup distilled water
1/8 cup witch hazel

****

Blend all the ingredients together in a food processor (make sure everything is blended well), and then strain. Use a cotton ball to apply to face.

Pineapple: Astringent, toner
Distilled water: Dilute
Witch hazel: astringent

Avoid the eye area

Remember to do your patch test.

****

Moisturizers

A Moisturizer is an emollient which coats the skin and forms a seal to protect the body's natural moisture. This makes the skin feel smoother and softer; reduces cracking and roughness.

None of the recipes are intended for internal use

Rose Milk Moisturizer
For Normal Skin

****

3 tablespoons rose water
1 tablespoon milk

****

Follow rose water recipe on page 87
Combine ingredients. Apply to face using a
cotton ball. Rinse with cool water.

Rose water: moisturizer
Milk: Cleanser, emollient

Avoid the eye area

Remember to do your patch test.

****

Orange Milk Moisturizer

For Normal- Oily Skin

****

2 tablespoon orange juice
3 tablespoons distilled water
1 tablespoon milk

****

Combine ingredients. Apply to face using a cotton ball. Rinse with cool water.

Orange juice: Astringent, toner
Distilled water: moisturizer
Milk: Cleanser, emollient, moisturizer

Avoid the eye area

Remember to do your patch test.

****

Aloe and Jojoba Moisturizer

For Normal- Oily Skin

****

2 tablespoon aloe vera gel
1 teaspoon jojoba oil

****

Combine ingredients. Apply to face using a
cotton ball. Rinse with cool water.

Aloe Vera: moisturizer
Jojoba oil: moisturizer

Avoid the eye area

Remember to do your patch test.

****

Jojoba Moisturizer

For Dry- Normal Skin

****

4 tablespoons jojoba oil
1 tablespoon distilled water
1 tablespoons grated beeswax

****

Combine ingredients. Apply to face using a
cotton ball. Rinse with cool water.

Jojoba oil: moisturizer
Distilled water: moisten
Bees wax: Emulsifier, softens

Avoid the eye area

Remember to do your patch test.

****

Sesame Moisturizer

For Dry-Skin

****

4 tablespoons sesame oil
2 tablespoons olive oil
1 tablespoon distilled water
2 tablespoons grated beeswax

****

Combine ingredients. Apply to face using a
cotton ball. Rinse with cool water.

Sesame oil: moisturizer
Olive oil: Softener, emollient
Distilled water: moisten
Bees wax: Emulsifier, softens

Avoid the eye area

Remember to do your patch test.

****

Glossary

****

Alfalfa sprouts: Astringent, soothes

Almonds: Exfoliant, emollient

Aloe Vera Gel: Greaseless moisturizer

Anti-inflammatory: A substance that reduces inflammation of the skin

Antiseptic: Substances that may kill, retard, or prevent the growth of bacteria

Apple: Dissolves facial oil, exfoliant also rich in vitamins A and C

Apple cider vinegar: Astringent, dissolves facial oil

Astringent: A toner and a refresher; temporarily reduces the size of pores

Avocado: Moiturizer, emollient, rich in vitamin E

Baking soda: Cleanser, skin softener and soother

Banana: Humectant and moisturizer high in potassium and vitamin C

Basil: Skin soother

****

Beer: *Skin soother, conditioner*

Bees wax: *Emulsifier, softens*

Cantaloupe: *Refresher, soother with vitamins A and C*

Carrot: *Antiseptic, cleaner, soother with vitamin A*

Chamomile: *Anti-inflammatory, soother, Healant*

Catnip: *Astringent, toner*

Cleanser: *A substance that loosens dirt and oils*

Cornmeal: *Exfoliant, absorbs excess oil*

Cornstarch: *Thickener, absorbs oil*

Cucumber: *Astringent, refresher*

Distilled water: *Has been purified by condensation and evaporation*

Egg: *Emulsifier contains protein*

Emollient: *An agent used to soothe and soften skin*

Emulsifier: *A material that binds two different materials together*

Exfoliant: *A material which aids in shedding dead skin cells and dirt*

****

Gelatin: A thickening agent

Grape: Anti-inflammatory, exfoliant

Grapefruit: Astringent, exfoliant

Healant: A substance that heals skin abrasions

Honey: Humectant, conditioner, emollient

Humectant: Slows the loss of moisture from the skin

Jojoba oil: Soother, Moisturizer

Lecithin: Emulsifier derived from soybean oil

Lemon: Astringent, toner oil remover

Lime: Astringent, refresher, exfoliant

Milk: Moisturizer, soother and emulsifier, mild cleanser, emollient

Mint: Stimulant

Moisturizer: An emollient which makes skin feel softer

Oats: Cleanser, soother

Olive oil: Softener, emollient

Orange: Astringent

Parsley: Cleanser, healant

****

Papaya: Exfoliant, skin conditioner

Peach: Conditioner, soother

Pineapple: Anti-inflammatory, exfoliant

Pine nuts: Conditioner, used as an exfoliant

Rosemary: astringent, stimulant

Rose Petals: skin softener, mild cleanser

Sage: Antiseptic, soother

Sesame seeds: Exfoliant, cleanser

Sesame oil: Moisturizer

Smoother: An ingredient that gives a more even texture to the skin

Soother: An ingredient that relieves pain on the skin

Soymilk: Softens, Moisturizer, soother

Stimulant: An agent that increases circulation

Strawberry: Astringent, conditioner, cleanser

Tomato: Astringent

Toner: A substance that tightens the skin.

Vodka: Astringent

Watermelon: Astringent, toner

****

Witch hazel: *Astringent*

Yogurt: *Soothing, helps restore ph balance*

Index

****

****

Grape and Cucumber Toner: 78

Grapefruit: 71, 87

Grapefruit Toner: 71

Honey: 4, 5, 6, 12, 13, 14, 16, 17, 18, 19, 20, 34, 37, 38, 39, 41, 42, 44, 45, 47, 48, 49, 50, 51, 52, 55, 56, 57, 59, 60, 89

Honey and Egg Mask: 34

Honey Cornmeal Scrub: 17

Honey Oat Scrub: 14

Jojoba Moisturizer: 84

Jojoba oil: 83, 84, 88

Lemon: 8, 11, 39, 43, 63, 65, 67, 69, 76, 88

Lemon and Egg Mask: 43

Lemon and Honey Mask: 39

Lemon and Apple Toner: 69

Lemon Facial Toner: 67

Lime: 66, 88

Lime Mint Toner: 66

Milk: 5, 7, 13, 17, 37, 40, 46, 65, 81, 82, 88

Milk and Honey Mask: 37

****

****

Peel off Mask: 40

Pest Mask: 60

Pesto Scrub: 18

Pineapple: 19, 79, 88

Pineapple Scrub: 19

Pineapple Toner: 79

Pine nuts: 11, 12, 18

Quickie Cleanser: 4

Quickie Wash: 3

Rose Milk Moisturizer: 81

Rose Rosemary Toner: 72

Rosemary: 30, 72, 89

Rosemary Steam: 30

Rose Petals: 24, 62, 72, 81, 89

Rose Petal Steam: 24

Rose Water: 62

Sage: 27, 89

Sage Steam: 27

Sesame Moisturizer: 85

****

****

****

Dawn M. Waldock

Printed in the United States
1419500001B/115